Cath Kidston®

THE LITTLE BOOK OF
HEALTH & HAPPINESS

Cath Kidston®

THE LITTLE BOOK OF HEALTH & HAPPINESS

101 ways to brighten up your day

Hardie Grant

QUADRILLE

INTRODUCTION

Ever since the first Cath Kidston shop opened its doors in London's Holland Park in 1993, our brand has been devoted to brightening up your day by using pretty, colourful prints with a nod to nostalgia to turn modern products into something witty, fresh and fun.

A brighter day means a happier, healthier day – and we firmly believe that a positive outlook is the best place to start. Little changes can make a big difference, so to help you on your way, we've compiled *Cath Kidston: The Little Book of Health & Happiness: 101 ways to brighten up your day.*

Whether you'd like to up your positivity, master a new yoga pose or simply prep a healthy packed lunch, on every page you'll find uplifting, inspirational tips paired with our unique prints to create a bible of brightness, just for you. Dip in for encouragement and a daily insight, or read it all in one go!

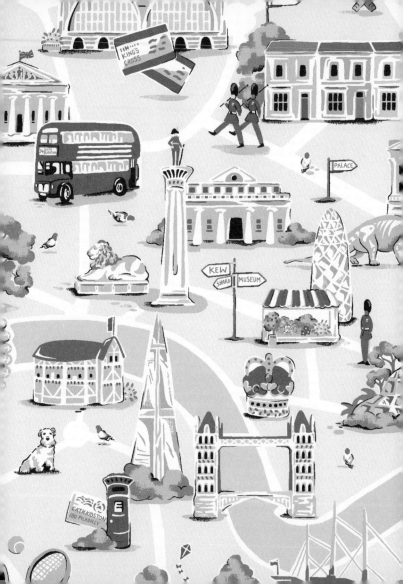

#1

STAY HYDRATED.

Drink more water! To keep things fresh, why not add a sprig of mint or a slice of lemon or cucumber to your glass?

#2

GO OFF GRID.

Take a day for a digital detox. Put your phone/laptop/tablet away — without the buzzing and beeping, you'll feel more peaceful and start to connect more with those around you.

#3

SET YOUR ALARM 10 MINUTES EARLIER THAN NORMAL.

It'll help reduce stress and you'll avoid the morning rush.

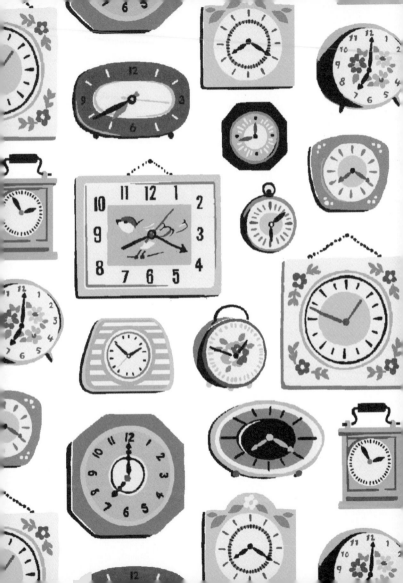

#4

JUST BREATHE.

When you're feeling stressed, give yourself a moment to close your eyes, sit up straight and focus on nothing but your breathing.

#5

GO FOR A BIKE RIDE.

Make the most of pedal power to explore a new part of town or take a trip out to the countryside. (We won't tell if you stop off for a cuppa along the way!)

#6

SMILE — IT'S CONTAGIOUS.

Turn that frown upside down. Each time you smile it's like a feel-good party in your brain, plus you'll find others are more likely to smile back at you too. Go ahead and share the happiness.

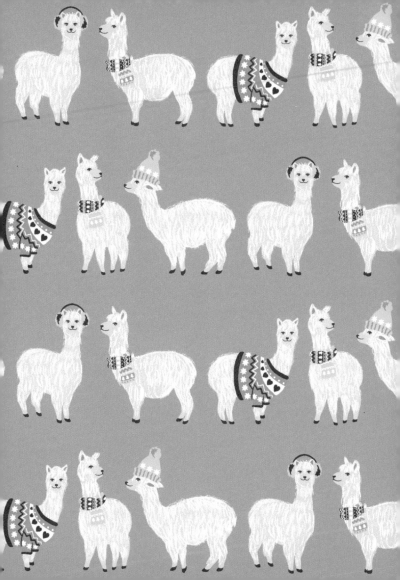

#7

PREPARE FOR THE
SNACK ATTACK.

Keep something healthy in your bag to snack on. Nuts,
bananas and apples are all portable, nutritious and filling.

#8

GET SOME GOALS.

A dream written down with a date becomes a goal, and a goal broken down into steps becomes a plan. Take half an hour to check in with yourself and write down five goals that you'd like to work towards, then reflect on the actions needed to accomplish them.

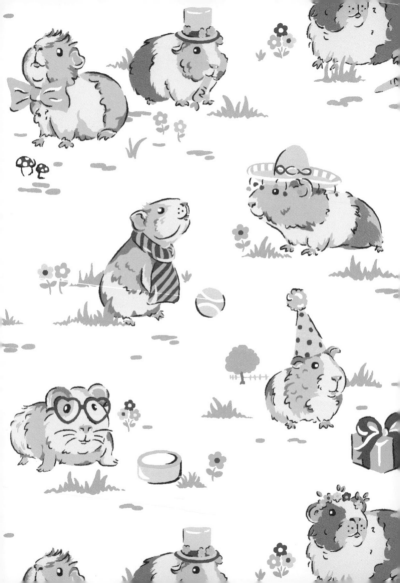

#9

LAUGHTER IS THE
BEST MEDICINE.

From a good giggle to a full-on belly laugh, a chuckle can do more than brighten up your day — it can help relieve physical tension and stress and have a positive impact on your health, too.

#10

START YOUR MORNING WITH A STRETCH.

Lie on your back and straighten out your legs.

Stretch your arms out to either side of your body and relax.

Swing your right leg over your left leg, twisting at the hip, and let the right leg lie at a 90° angle.

Ensure your shoulders remain flat on the bed/floor and turn your head to look in the opposite direction to the bent leg.

Take two to four long and deep breaths, relaxing on each exhale.

Repeat on the other side.

#11

PREPARE A HEALTHY LUNCH THE NIGHT BEFORE.

Homemade lunches are a great way to save money and use up last night's leftovers. To serve in style, why not pack them up in one of our pretty printed lunch boxes?

#12

HAVE AN EVENING IN.

Staying in is the new going out! Light some candles and
snuggle under a blanket with your favourite film or book.

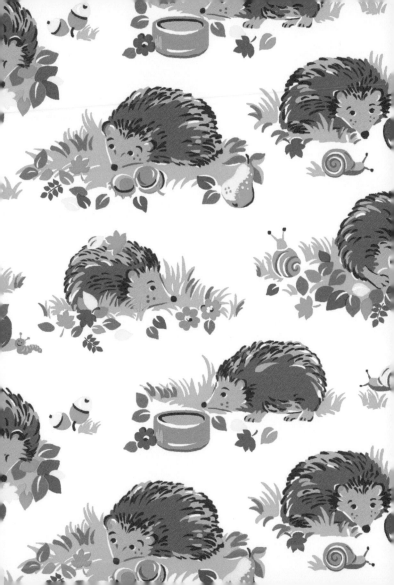

#13

CREATE A POSITIVE
PLAYLIST.

Compile the songs that make you feel happy and motivated
into one playlist. Then, when you're feeling blue,
you know what to do!

#14

HAVE A CLEAR-OUT.

Turn all the hanging clothes in your wardrobe around so the hangers are facing the wrong way. Every time you take something out to wear, replace it with the hanger back in its correct position. After a few weeks, you'll see what you don't wear — then it's time for a trip to the charity shop!

#16

PAUSE.

Make yourself a cup of tea in your favourite mug and take a mindful moment to stop and reflect on what you have achieved today.

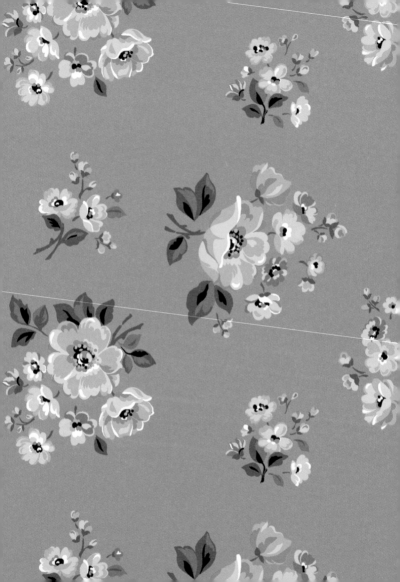

#17

START EACH DAY WITH
A GRATEFUL HEART.

As you get up, think of five things you're grateful for and
write them down in a notebook. By the end of the week,
you'll have a long list of why life is wonderful!

#18

ENJOY YOUR FOOD.

You've got to nourish to flourish! Eat mindfully and think about creating healthy eating habits rather than restrictions.

#19

GET A GYM BUDDY.

Fitness can be fun! Teaming up will help keep you motivated and accountable — meaning you're more likely to make that morning workout!

#20

READ SOMETHING NEW.

Even if it's not what you'd usually go for, give it a try.
You never know what treasure you may discover!

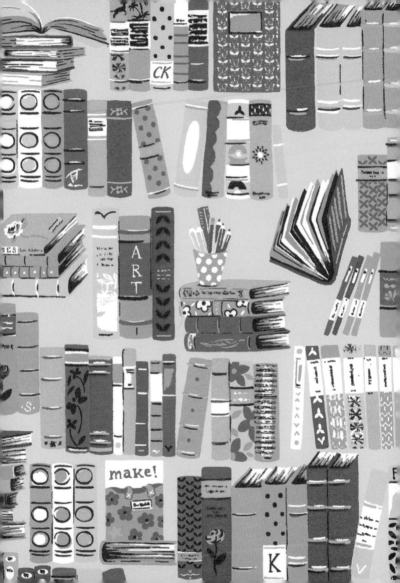

#21

CLEAR MIND CLUTTER.

Note down your to-do list to free up valuable mental space. Once it's on paper, you'll find it's easier to order and prioritise your responsibilities. Plus, when a task is done, you get to tick it off!

#22

BLOW AWAY THE COBWEBS.

Embrace the invigoration of a windy day. Wrap up warm
and climb a hill, then stand facing the wind. Let the
briskness of the breeze blow away your worries!

#23

EXPRESS YOURSELF.

Share how you feel with your nearest and dearest —
don't forget to tell them how much they mean to you!

#24

FUEL UP FOR THE DAY.
TURKISH EGGS ON TOAST (Serves 2)

150g/5½oz Greek yoghurt
½ a very small garlic clove, crushed
2 large slices poppy seed bloomer
35g/1½oz butter

2 eggs
1 heaped teaspoon Turkish chilli flakes
6 small sage leaves
flaky sea salt

Bring a pan of water to a simmer. Spoon the yoghurt into a bowl, add the crushed garlic and plenty of salt and beat together. Toast the bread. Melt the butter in a small frying pan. While the butter is melting, gently crack the eggs into the simmering water and poach for 2–3 minutes. Once the butter has started to foam, stir in the chilli flakes and sage leaves and let them sizzle for a few seconds. Drizzle a little butter over each slice of toast then spoon the yoghurt on top. Lift the eggs out of the water and drain, then place on top of the yoghurt. Drizzle over the chilli and sage butter and eat straight away.

#25

GIVE YOURSELF A BREAK.

Don't feel like it? That's ok! Listen to your body
and take some time to relax.

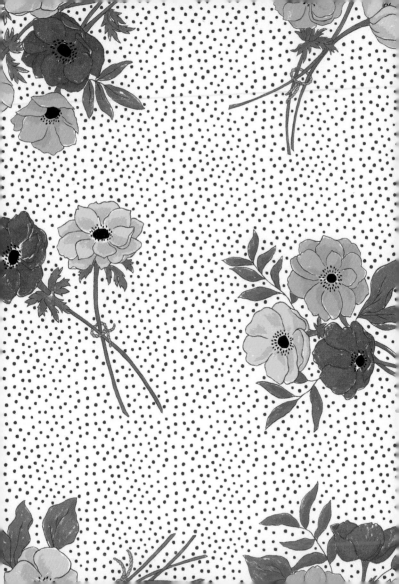

#26

DETOX YOUR BOUDOIR.

Your bedroom is a sanctuary, so keep it a phone/tablet/laptop/TV free zone. You'll improve your sleep quality while you're at it.

#27

EXPLORE MORE.

Take a day for yourself and be a tourist in your local town or city.
Discover secret pockets of green or stop for a coffee at a
café you've never tried before.

#28

REMEMBER, IT'S OK
TO SAY NO.

Whether it's because you don't have time, or you'd rather
relax than go out, give yourself permission to say
'no' without feeling guilty or selfish.

#29

SILENCE THE INNER CRITIC.

Get into the habit of talking to yourself as you would a friend.
Be positive and encouraging — don't bring yourself down!

#30

GET FIT AND ORGANISED.

Invest in a stylish yet functional sports bag, then organise your kit before hitting the gym. It'll help save time and energy for where it counts – your workout!

#31

SURPRISE YOURSELF — SPONTANEITY IS THE FIRST STEP ON THE ROAD TO ADVENTURE!

#32

GET CRAFTY.

Unleash your inner creative streak and have a go at making something from scratch. Whether it's knitting a scarf, sewing a cushion or building a set of shelves, find something that you enjoy!

#33

THINK POSITIVE WHEN THE GOING GETS TOUGH.

Remember, everything happens for a reason. Life, like nature, moves in cycles so if you're going through a rough patch, take heart and know it will pass. Tomorrow is a new, brighter day!

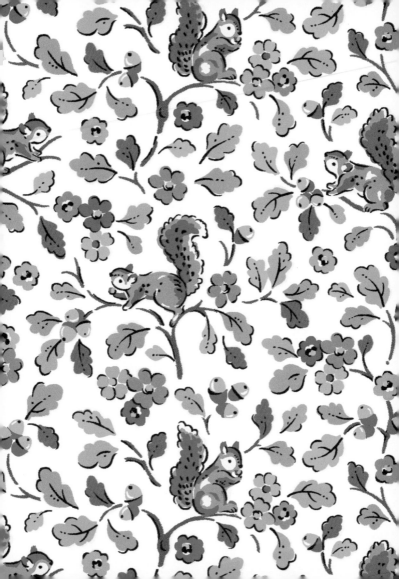

#34

DARE TO DAYDREAM.

Allow yourself time every day to let your mind wander.
It's good for the soul!

#35

EXERCISE YOUR BRAIN.

Puzzle books, riddles, quizzes and crosswords are all ways to exercise your brain, but you can also set yourself mini challenges. Simple things like remembering your shopping list or recalling a favourite journey in your mind will help keep your brain in tip top condition.

KNOW YOUR FATS.
GUACAMOLE (Medium-size dip)

2 avocados

1 lime, zest and juice

1 garlic clove, minced

1 teaspoon chilli flakes

½ teaspoon smoked paprika

handful fresh coriander, finely chopped

handful fresh mint, finely chopped

salt and pepper, to taste

Mash the avocado in a bowl then stir in all the other ingredients. Serve on toast with poached eggs or with a Mexican feast!

Good fats (polyunsaturated fatty acids and monounsaturated fats) eaten in moderation help lower cholesterol and reduce the risk of heart disease. These 'heart happy' fats can be found in avocados, olive oil, coconut oil, sardines and salmon.

#37

USE THE MAGIC WORDS.

Don't forget to say 'please' and 'thank you' often.

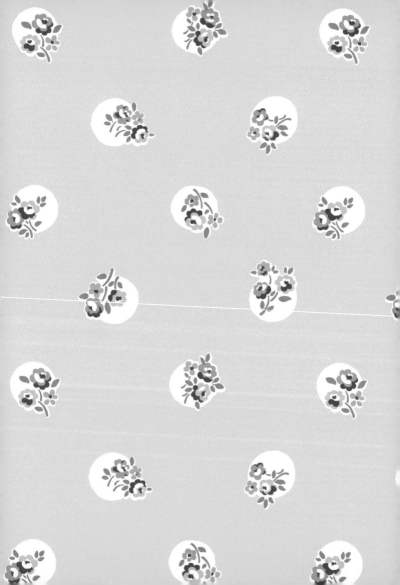

#38

FIND YOUR RHYTHM.

Choose an upbeat track that gives you a happy vibe and
pop it on first thing in the morning. Hello sunshine!

#39

PAMPER POWER.

Take a long, luxurious soak in the bath with your favourite lotions, potions and candles. Add a couple of drops of lavender essential oil to help you relax.

#40

STRIKE A POSE.

Power posing is an easy way to boost confidence and it can even help you tackle daunting tasks. Stand tall, feet apart, chest out, shoulders back and hands on your hips – just like a superhero.

#41

TAKE A CAT NAP.

Make like our furry friends and rest when you feel the need.
Listen to your body and top up on those zzz's. An afternoon nap
can be just enough to restore energy and enthusiasm.

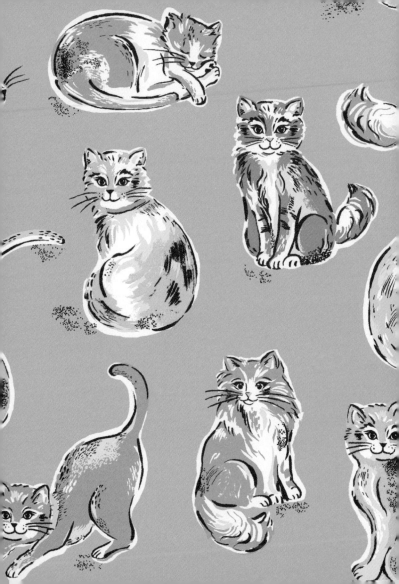

#42

BRIGHTEN YOUR MOOD BY INJECTING SOME COLOUR INTO YOUR WARDROBE.

Wear red for a positive, confident 'can-do' attitude. Go all the way with a head-to-toe ensemble, or opt for a subtle splash of colour with accessories like scarves, jewellery or a vibrant handbag.

#43

WATCH THE SUN RISE, AND
LOOK FORWARD TO A NEW DAY.

#44

APPRECIATE THE LITTLE THINGS.

Go for a walk and explore your surroundings. Leave your phone and music at home, and try to absorb all the things you can see, hear, smell and touch. Take everything in, from the rustle of the leaves to the sound of the birds in the trees.

#45

INDULGE YOURSELF.

Every once in a while, enjoy a simple treat like going out for tea and cake with friends. Pleasure is multiplied when you share it with others.

#46

BE FLEXIBLE FROM HEAD TO TOE.

Take up yoga, which will help look after your mind
as well as your muscles.

#47

FEED YOUR GUT.
MISO AUBERGINE (Side dish)

1 aubergine
1 tablespoon sesame oil
1 tablespoon miso paste
sesame seeds

Slice the aubergine lengthways into half-centimetre slices. Brush both sides of each slice with sesame oil and miso paste. Place into a hot griddle pan and cook for around 6 minutes on each side. Sprinkle with sesame seeds before serving.

Include probiotics in your diet by choosing foods like sauerkraut, kefir, miso, yoghurt, kombucha and pickles.

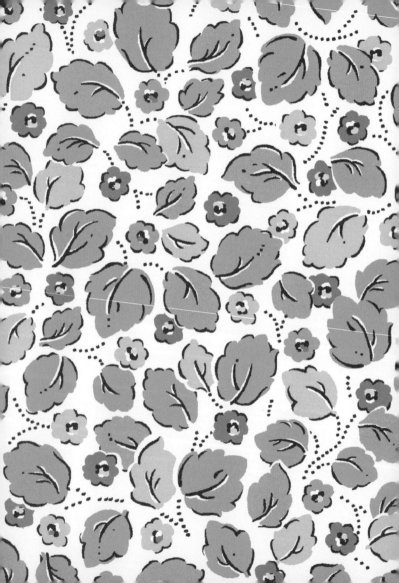

#48

SEE THE SEASONS.

Whether it's the gold of autumn, the green of summer or the frost of winter, take a moment to get outside and revel in the glory of nature.

#49

WATCH THE SUN SET.

It's proof that endings can be beautiful.

#50

SAY WELL DONE TO YOU.

Make a list of all your successes. Start with small daily achievements,
then move on to bigger goals. Read through each one, and remember
how it felt when you attained them. Add to the list each week,
then reflect on it at the end of the year and you'll see just
how far you've come!

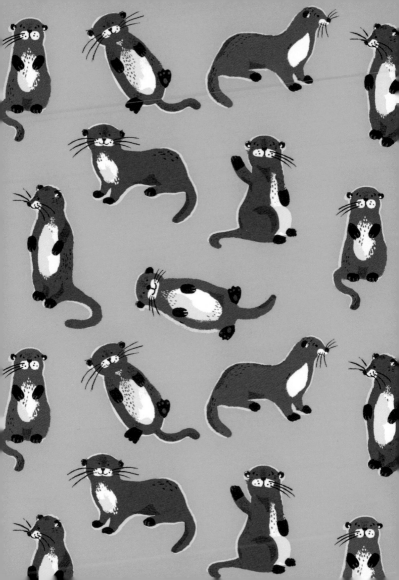

#52

HUG IT OUT.

Share a hug! Hugs boost levels of oxytocin, the 'happy hormone' which promotes feelings of contentment, helping reduce stress and anxiety.

#53

TAKE TIME TO DO WHAT MAKES YOU HAPPY.

#54

FORGET THE MISTAKE.

Remember the lesson.

#55

UP YOUR FIVE A DAY AND PUT A SPRING IN YOUR STEP.

SUPER SMOOTHIE

1 banana
handful blueberries
handful strawberries

handful spinach
1 teaspoon honey
2 tablespoons natural yoghurt

Place all the ingredients into a blender and pulse until smooth. Loosen with a little milk if it's too thick. Pour into a glass and enjoy!

#56

EMBRACE FLOWER POWER.

Think floral and add some colour to your home. From bloom-inspired furnishings and accessories, to displays of your favourite flowers, lift your spirits and bring the outside in.

#57

**FACE YOUR FEAR — REPEAT
'I CAN DO THIS' UNTIL YOU CAN.**

#58

WRITE A JOURNAL.

Keep a record and store those golden moments. Find a notebook you like and fill it full of mementos, quotes and reminders of special times.

#59

INHALE, EXHALE.

Take a minute to focus on your breathing.

As you inhale, extend the breath for one slow count,
then do the same as you exhale.

Repeat this, and extend the breath one more time.

As your breathing slows and you take in more air,
you'll feel instantly revitalised.

#61

STOP THINKING OF WHAT COULD GO WRONG. THINK OF WHAT COULD GO RIGHT.

#62

GET GREEN FINGERED.

Purchase a new cactus or house plant. Watch as the plant grows and develops over time. If it produces off-shoots, propagate them and share one with a friend.

#63

ROAR LIKE A DINOSAUR.

Imagine you're purging yourself of all frustrations. Throw your head back, take a deep breath and let out a mighty roar. It's an instant stress buster!

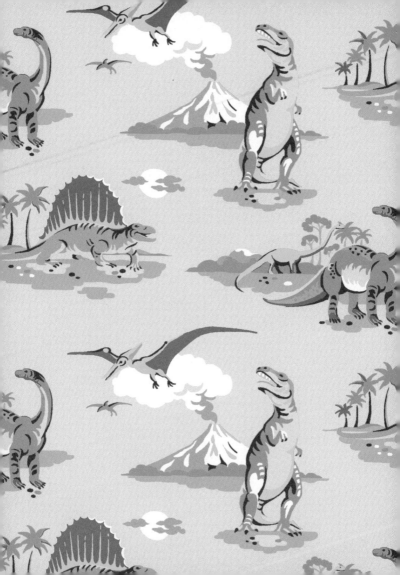

#64

BE KIND, TO YOURSELF AND OTHERS.

#65

FOLLOW YOUR NOSE.

Smells can lift our spirits and remind us of special memories.
Experiment with scent and find fragrances you love. From perfumed
candles to essential oils, fill your home with lovely aromas that make
you feel happy.

#66

DON'T LET THE WEATHER DAMPEN YOUR DAY.

There's nothing like splashing through puddles, so get your waterproofs and wellies on and go for a stroll on a grey day.

#67

TRY A NEW RECIPE.

What's cooking, good looking? Look to the internet for inspiration or borrow a book from a friend — let the pages fall open to a recipe and have a go!

#68

GREET THE SUN.

In the morning, on rising, open the curtains and stand tall.

Throw your arms wide open to embrace the sun.

Stretch your spine gently and roll on to your tiptoes, then slowly lower yourself back down and wrap your arms around your body.

#69

GET STRONG.

Whether you hit the gym or grab a couple of cans of soup for bicep curls, incorporate some weight training into your normal exercise routine. It helps strengthen your muscles and protect your bones as well as improve your ability to perform activities in daily life.

#70

GO BIRD WATCHING.

Take a walk through your local park and look up into the trees.
Spend some time quietly watching, and you'll see and hear a
host of different birds. Take a cute notebook with you so
that you can mark down what you've seen.

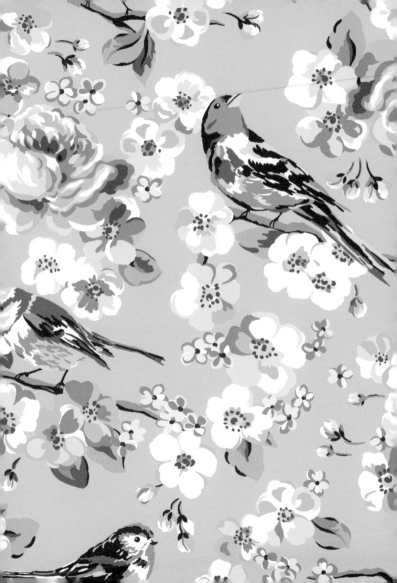

#71

TIDY DESK = TIDY MIND.

Organise paperwork and get rid of excess rubbish, then treat yourself
to some pretty new stationery so you can work in style.

#72

GRAB A HAIRBRUSH AND SING
YOUR HEART OUT. YOU ARE
A SUPERSTAR!

#73

RECONNECT WITH AN OLD FRIEND.

Say hello to someone you've lost touch with and find out what they've been up to. It's never too late to rekindle a friendship.

#74

DON'T WAIT FOR THE PERFECT MOMENT.

Take the moment and make it perfect.

#75

TAKE A TRIP TO THE COAST AND BREATHE IN THE SEA AIR.

Whatever the weather, stroll along the beach and take in the view.
Watch the waves and indulge in a spot of beach-combing
while you're there.

TRUST YOUR INTUITION.

Notice any niggling feelings in your stomach and understand the difference between nervous excitement and anxiety. When something feels right, go for it. When something feels wrong, pause and think.

#77

WELCOME A
FOUR-LEGGED FRIEND.

If you can't have a dog of your own, borrow one! Go on long walks and enjoy the benefits of man's best friend.

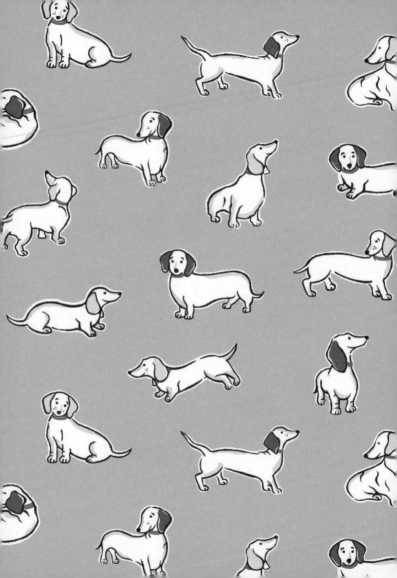

#78

ENJOY SOME RETAIL THERAPY.

Money doesn't buy happiness, but that doesn't mean you can't enjoy splurging occasionally — you deserve it after all! Next time you buy something for yourself, why not pick up something for a friend too? Surprise presents are the best presents.

#79

JAZZ UP LONG JOURNEYS.

Create the perfect road trip playlist and fill up a pretty floral flask
with a batch of hot chocolate or tea.

#80

LEND A HAND.

Whether it's assisting a neighbour by doing some gardening or shopping for them, or offering to work at a local charity shop, never underestimate the power of a helping hand.

#81

HAVE A TEA PARTY.

Bring your friends together over tea and cake —
it's the perfect way to have a relaxed catch up!

#82

BE COOL.

Feeling hot? Hold each wrist under the cold tap for a minute and focus on how the chilly water feels against your skin.

#83

LEAVE WORK AT WORK.

Set clear boundaries between work and personal life, so you
can switch off and enjoy time with friends and family.

PLANT BEE-FRIENDLY FLOWERS AND PLANTS IN YOUR GARDEN.

Dog roses, honeysuckle, snapdragons, lavender and hyacinth
are all bee favourite blooms.

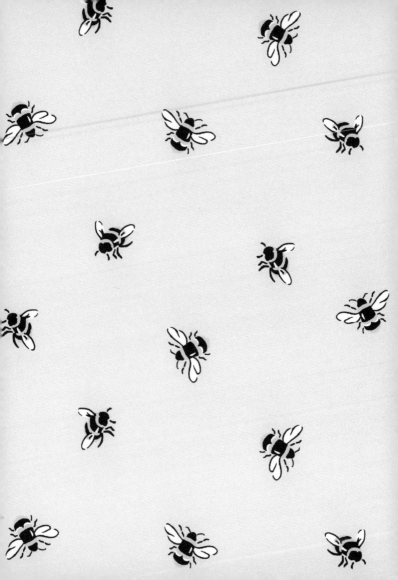

#85

TURN OFF THE TV.

One night a week, switch the box off and choose a board game instead — it's the ideal way to bring laughter (and a bit of friendly competition) back to family life.

#86

CREATE A PERSONAL POWER MANTRA.

Start by deciding how you'd like to feel then, once you have a sense of it in your mind, turn it into a declarative statement. For example, if you want to feel more energised, your mantra might be 'In taking this time to be calm, I am rebooting my energy levels'. Repeat the mantra in your head, or out loud as often as you can throughout the day.

#87

INHALE THE FUTURE.
EXHALE THE PAST.

Take some time each day for a spot of meditation.

#88

TRY SOMETHING NEW.

Choose something you've always wanted to try and make it your new hobby. You'll learn new skills, meet people with similar interests and have a great time while doing it.

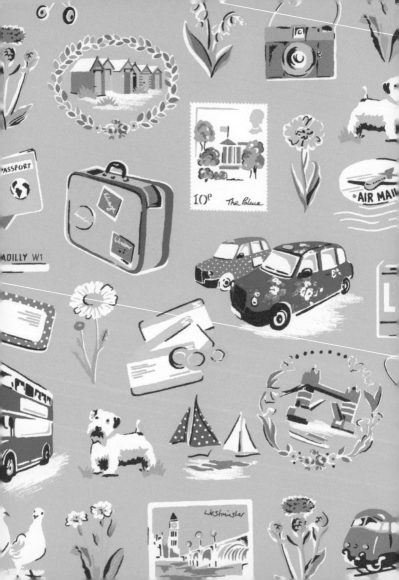

#89

PICNICS AREN'T JUST FOR THE SUMMER.

Make the most of each season and try a picnic during autumn and winter. Wrap up warm, take a flask of homemade soup or a stew packed full of seasonal veg, and enjoy the beauty of the changing landscape.

#90

INCREASE THE NUMBER OF STEPS YOU TAKE EACH DAY.

Get off the bus/tram/tube a stop earlier, or walk to and from work. And remember — always take the stairs.

#91

LET IT GO.

When a worry arises, ask yourself 'can I do anything about this?'. If the answer is yes, take action. If it's no, take a deep breath and let it go. You can't do anything to influence the situation, so relax and release your anxiety.

#92

HAVE DOS INSTEAD OF DON'TS.

When tackling bad habits, don't create a list of strict rules. Instead be positive and think of things you can do! For example, rather than cutting things out of your diet, make the decision to eat more fruit and vegetables.

#93

LET LIFE SURPRISE YOU.

Resist the urge to control events. Let life surprise you with
a curveball and allow new adventures to unfold.

#94

REMEMBER, ANYTHING IS POSSIBLE!

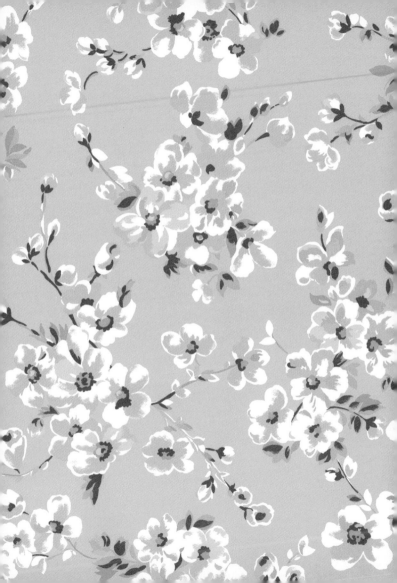

#95

FIND A MENTOR.

Choose someone you admire and identify with – this could be a friend, colleague, or even someone in the media that inspires you. Make a list of the attributes that you admire about this person and think of ways that you can develop these strengths.

#96

BELIEVE IN YOURSELF.

In order to succeed, you must first believe you can.

#97

RECYCLE AND UPCYCLE.

Give items a new lease of life, either by passing
them on or re-vamping them.

#98

UPGRADE YOUR ZZZ'S.

Get into a routine of going to bed and getting up at the same time every day. This helps settle your body clock. Plus, be sure to keep your room dark, well ventilated and free of any tech or work-related paraphernalia.

#99

LIVE SIMPLY.
DREAM BIG.
BE GRATEFUL.
GIVE LOVE.
LAUGH LOTS.

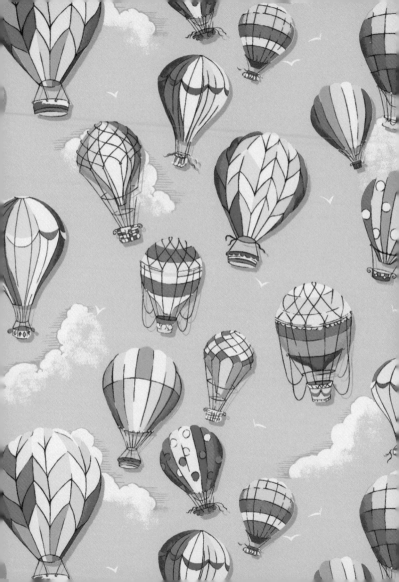

#100

BOOST YOUR ENERGY LEVELS AND IMMUNE SYSTEM.

Increase your intake of magnesium with leafy greens, seeds, beans, wholegrains and nuts, or even treat yourself to some dark chocolate!

#101

BE YOURSELF AT ALL TIMES, IN ALL THINGS. YOU ARE BRILLIANT, LOVABLE AND UNIQUE!

Cath Kidston acknowledgements:
Andrea Yorston, Suzi Avens, Christine
Hafsten, Sue Chidler, Rebecca Hadley,
Helena Hunter Wood, Dominica Dudzuik,
Amber Morgan, Nicole Gray, Katie
Buckingham, Xenia Xenophontos,
Sarah Mulligan, Jen Inglis, Natasha
Hinds-Payne, Jack Weaver

For more Cath Kidston products,
visit cathkidston.com

Publishing Director: Sarah Lavelle
Editor: Harriet Butt
Editorial Assistant: Harriet Webster
Designer: Gemma Hayden
Words: Alison Davies
Production Director: Vincent Smith
Production Controller: Nikolaus Ginelli

Published in 2018 by Quadrille,
an imprint of Hardie Grant Publishing

Quadrille
52–54 Southwark Street
London SE1 1UN
quadrille.com

Cataloguing in Publication Data:
a catalogue record for this book is
available from the British Library.

Text, design and layout © Quadrille 2018
Illustrations © Cath Kidston 2018

Reprinted in 2018, 2020 (twice)
10 9 8 7 6 5 4

ISBN 978 178713 252 8
CK ISBN 978 178713 320 4

Printed in China

MIX
Paper from
responsible sources
FSC® C020056
www.fsc.org